The Ultimate Paleo Diet Cookbook

More Than 80 Recipes That Are Designed to Be Easy and Quick to Prepare, with a Focus on Nutrient-Dense Ingredients

Written by

Robert Kaveman

Table Of Contents

Introduction

All About the Paleo Diet

Why to Try a Paleo Diet ?

All it takes to keep up with the latest diet is a quick look at the magazines.

These days, there is a new diet every week. They always promise weight loss and improved health. But many of these diets are not based on scientific truth and any results from them fade quickly too.

One good diet is called the Paleo diet.

It can help people lose weight or improve their digestion, or even just make them healthier in general.

The Paleo diet is a special diet for people who are interested in eating what early humans ate.

You don't have to hunt or look for food, but certain rules apply.

This diet excludes processed carbs and refined sugars as well as dairy products, grains, and legumes.

After you get used to this diet you will be feeling better than if you are on the standard Western Diet.

What is the Paleo Diet?

There are lots of diets that promise amazing results. But many of them don't work or, if they do, the results only last for a short time.

The paleo diet is different because it is a healthy lifestyle that involves eating mostly natural foods that have not been changed by man.

The name of the paleo diet comes from the Paleolithic Era when humans lived without farming and hunted animals for food.

People in the past did not have agriculture, so they hunted and gathered food. They ate from the land.

The Paleolithic Diet is like this too. People believe that our genetics (in other words, how our bodies work) has not changed since the time of hunting and gathering food from the land.

So we need to eat what is natural like animals, vegetables, fruits, nuts and seeds that are still around now too.

The paleo diet has been around for 40 years. It is popular now. People think it is new because it used to not be popular, but it's not new.

Following the paleo diet may not require you to hunt for your own food, but it does mean that you will need to think about what foods you are eating more carefully.

This diet focuses on proteins, fruit and vegetables, nuts and seeds. It also doesn't include processed foods or any dairy products.

Basically, the Paleo diet includes foods that are from the Paleolithic Era. This is before people had farms. It is a little bit flexible, but it is mostly about eating like they did then.

In 1975, a doctor named Dr. Walter Voegtlin published a book called The Stone Age Diet. In the book, he talked about how he treated patients with his diet that was like what people ate in the Paleolithic era.

He said that people with Crohn's disease and irritable bowel syndrome saw improvements in their health when they followed his diet which included eating large quantities of animal fats and proteins and very small quantities of carbohydrates.

Unfortunately, The Stone Age Diet did not go over well with the public. At that time, almost everyone thought you should only eat a low-fat and low-calorie diet.

Paleo Diet is an "Ancient" Diet but Good for Our "Modern" Times

After ten years, Dr. S. Boyd Eaton and Dr. Melvin Konner published a paper in The New England Journal of Medicine about the Paleo diet that helped support Dr. Voegtlin's research and got lots of attention from doctors and the media.

After their paper, they wrote a book called The Paleolithic Prescription: A Program of Diet & Exercise and a Design for Living which established the basic principles that most variations of the Paleo diet follow today.

The book explains why our Paleolithic ancestors ate a healthy diet. It is for modern times, so it will be easy to eat like them. They have lots of good information that shows the nutritional content of their diet and how to get that from today's food.

There are many versions of the Paleo diet. They are different in how strict they are and how much they follow the eating patterns of our Paleolithic ancestors.

This version is a more strict one that tries to be as close to what it would be like if we lived back then, but without being too difficult or complicated.

The Paleo diet is a good way to lose weight and be healthier. You do not have to change your whole lifestyle or spend time looking for things that you can't find. This diet is moderate, but it will work great.

The Paleo diet is a way of eating that replicates what our ancestors ate before agriculture. There are some people who literally hunt, gather, and forage all their food, but most people do not have the motivation or time to do this.

Fortunately, we can achieve the same results with food that we buy in stores and at farmers markets.

The Paleo diet is a type of food pyramid. On the top, you have meat and eggs. Then fats from plants, and then fruits and vegetables. At the bottom, you have nuts and seeds.

The opposite of what was recommended by USDA (United States Department of Agriculture).

The paleo diet is about eating good food like healthy meat, fresh fruit and vegetables. The paleo diet also includes things that are healthy, like nuts and seeds.

These foods are also in the Mediterranean Diet and the DASH Diet.

Though many people might think the paleo diet is restrictive, it is actually simpler to follow than you may think. You need to cut out all grains and dairy products, but that still leaves you with lots of options.

We will go into more detail about what foods are allowed on the paleo diet very soon but for now, let's just focus on how beneficial it can be.

The foods you eat on the paleo diet may be similar to any other diet that is based around healthy, natural food.

This is a list of the top benefits:

a) **More lean, and therefore more healthy, muscle mass**

The paleo diet is a diet that is about eating lean protein. This includes things like grass-fed meat, free-run poultry, and wild-caught fish. These would help you to build and maintain muscle mass.

b) **Paleo benefits improve digestive health**

Refined sugars and processed carbohydrates can cause inflammation in the intestinal tract. This is bad for your body because you won't be able to digest or get nutrition from the food that you eat. If you don't have these foods, your digestive system will start to heal.

c) Living longer and healthier lives

Following a diet low in processed foods and saturated fat will help you to live longer. It also helps you to avoid diseases that might shorten your life, so it is worth the change.

d) The Paleo diet consists of food high in concentrated nutrition

The foods in the paleo diet are rich in nutrients. Processed food is less rich in nutrients than natural food.

e) A Paleo diet is often recommended for those who suffer from allergies because it contains only real food

The paleo diet is not full of grains like corn and wheat. It also does not have dairy products.

f) It reduces inflammation

Inflammation is a problem that causes many diseases. The paleo diet has foods that can help from inflammation.

g) The Paleo diet increases energy levels

When you cut out foods that are bad for your digestive system, you can get better. When your digestion gets better, and when you start to absorb nutrients again, then you will have more energy.

h) A Paleo diet is often an effective way to lose weight

Though the paleo diet is not low in calories, it still helps you lose weight. It also has many foods that are high in nutrients and low in calories. This diet can help you lose weight and keep it off.

i) Eating a Paleo diet might reduce your risk for several diseases

Many of the most serious chronic diseases are related to food. They can happen because of an unhealthy diet. If you eat better food, then you might avoid these diseases.

The paleo diet is a very good way to have stable blood sugar levels. You don't eat sugar and carbohydrate foods when you are on the diet.

When your blood sugar is stable, your body can heal itself from insulin resistance and then you can digest food again.

A paleo diet can help you to maintain a healthy weight which will help prevent diabetes from coming back.

Keep reading to learn about the specific foods of the paleo diet.

The paleo diet has foods that are natural. It includes lean meats, poultry, eggs, fish and vegetables. The diet also has nuts, seeds and healthy fats.

The paleo diet is based on food that hasn't been altered by people. It includes lean proteins like beef and chicken but also fruits and vegetables.

This diet also includes nuts, seeds, and healthy fats. Refined sugars and processed carbohydrates are not good for the paleo diet. They cannot be eaten, nor can dairy products, grains, legumes or white potatoes.

The Paleo diet is a type of diet where you eat healthy foods. It can be effective because it is not just about what you eat, but also what you don't eat.

One part of the Paleo plan is to change the proportions and types of food that you eat, like avoiding processed foods, alcohol, grains, legumes and sugar.

To help you see which foods are allowed and which aren't on the paleo diet, here are some lists.

Proteins

Bacon	Beef	Bison	Chicken	Clams	Duck
Eggs	Elk	Fish	Goose	Lamb	Lobster
Pheasant	Pork	Quail	Rabbit	Scallops	Shrimp
Turkey	Venison	Veal			

Fruits and Vegetables

Apples	Apricots	Asparagus	Artichoke	Arugula	Bananas
Beets	Bell peppers	Bok choy	Blackberries	Blueberries	Broccoli
Brussels	Cabbage	Carrots	Carrots	Cantaloupe	Cauliflower
Celery	Cherries	Cucumber	Eggplant	Grapes	Grapefruit
Green beans	Guava	Herbs	Honeydew	Kale	Kohlrabi
Kiwi	Lemon	Lime	Lettuce	Leeks	Mango
Mushrooms	Nectarines	Onions	Papaya	Parsnips	Peaches
Pears	Pineapple	Plum	Pomegranate	Pumpkin	Raspberries
Spinach	Sprouts	Strawberries	Sweet potato	Swiss chard	Squash
Tomatoes	Turnips	Watermelon	Zucchini		

Nuts and Seeds

Almonds	Brazil nuts	Cashews	Chestnuts	Chia seeds
Flaxseeds	Hazelnuts	Hemp seeds	Macadamia nuts	Pecans
Pine nuts	Pumpkin seeds	Sesame seeds	Turkey	Walnuts

Healthy Fats

Avocados	Coconut oil	Ghee	Grass-fed butter	Lard
Macadamia oil	Olive oil	Tallow	Walnut oil	

Other Foods

Almond flour	Almond milk	Arrowroot powder	Baking powder	Baking soda
Cocoa powder	Coconut	Coconut aminos	Coconut flour	Coconut milk
Coffee	Dark chocolate	Honey	Maple syrup	Pepper
Salt	Spices	Stevia	Tapioca starch	Tea
Vanilla extract	Vinegar			

Fruits, Drinks and Vegetables

Alcohol	Artificial sweetners	Baked goods	Barley	Beans
Bread	Brown rice	Brown sugar	Candy	Canola oil
Cereal	Cheese	Chickpeas	Corn	Corn oil
Cornstarch	Couscous	Cow's milk	Cream cheese	Energy drinks
Ice cream	Lentils	Margarine	Oats	Pasta
Peanut butter	Peanuts	Quinoa	Regular yogurt	Rye
Soft drinks	Soy beans	Soy sauce	Split peas	Vegetable oil
Wheat	White potatoes	White rice	White sugar	

Note: This list is not complete. Avoid all grains, dairy products, and legumes as well as processed foods and refined sugars.

Meats, Eggs and Seafood

This food group is where you will find most of your calories. All types of meat, fish, shellfish, and eggs are allowed. But there are guidelines for choosing the right foods.

The most important thing is to choose high quality foods and make sure that they are prepared with Paleo-approved ingredients.

Fats from Plant Sources

You can get fats from olives and avocadoes. Nuts also provide fat. Butter is a dairy product so it should not be used in cooking or preparing foods.

Use olive oil for cooking and grapeseed oil or extra virgin olive oil for uncooked dressings.

Nuts and Seeds

Nuts and seeds are from the Paleolithic-era. All nuts are allowed, but peanuts which are a legume.

Seeds are also allowed, including flax seeds, sunflower seeds, pumpkin seeds, sesame seeds and others.

If you want pasta and rice, quinoa is also okay because it is a seed and it can be eaten just like rice or pasta.

Fruits and Vegetables

The fruits that are allowed on the Paleo diet are those that were easy to find before people started farming. These include berries like cranberries, raspberries, strawberries and blueberries.

Tree fruits like apples, peaches, plums, cherries and nectarines also count as fruit.

Pick vegetables from the ground. This will be vegetables that you cannot grow. This includes potatoes, sweet potatoes, carrots and parsnips, but also includes wild vegetables such as lettuces and leafy greens. These vegetables include tomatoes, peppers, squash and zucchini.

Condiments

You can have some condiments, but make sure they don't have sugar. Also, try to use herbs and spices instead of condiments.

For example, ketchup is not allowed because it has sugar in it; mustard is okay because it does not usually have sugar added to it.

Beverages

You should drink water and unsweetened juices. You should not have too much of these. You can't drink other drinks, like tea, coffee, alcohol or wine.

Some recipes in this cookbook call for organic wine because it does not contain sulfites or other additives.

Processed Foods

Do not eat fast food, frozen meals or store-bought sweets and snacks.

Grains

Grains are grown and then made into food. Grains can be used to make bread, pasta, rice, oats, and barley.

You should not eat these grains if you want to have a pre-agricultural diet.

Legumes

As with grains, legumes such as beans, peas, soy and soy derivatives are not good for you.

They are agricultural products and therefore they are off-limits.

Sugar

The Paleo diet can change your blood sugar levels.

It may also help you to avoid getting diabetes or metabolic syndrome.

That's because on the Paleo diet, you don't eat sugars.

Artificial sweeteners are not necessary, but honey is okay in moderation and dark chocolate is okay too.

A paleo diet is a lifestyle rather than just a dietary choice, and there are many benefits you get from it.

One of the hardest skills in becoming more paleo-oriented at home, for example, is to stomach your food.

Here are some tips on how to make this process easier:

Start eating more protein and less carbohydrates. Eat a moderate amount of healthy fats, too.

At each meal, put some vegetables on your plate. Have grains and legumes with the vegetables instead of fruits.

Cook your food with coconut oil or olive oil. Do not eat too much of any type of saturated fat.

Use natural sweeteners like honey and maple syrup instead of granulated sugar and brown sugar.

Focus on cooking methods that are healthy, like baking, grilling and poaching.

As you change your diet, you will find that it is not so hard to follow the paleo diet.

When you go grocery shopping, take this list of food with you and buy only what is on the list.

Generally, the foods in the outer aisles of grocery stores are safe. For example, fresh produce, meat and seafood.

If you want to eat paleo foods, you should stop buying any food that is not paleo.

Then buy as many approved foods as you need so that you have plenty of options to choose from.

Just because you're on the paleo diet doesn't mean that you can't enjoy food.

You can use fresh herbs and dried spices to add flavor to your favorite dishes.

You also can go out to eat, but might have to order a dish that isn't what you are used to ordering.

Some dishes at the restaurant are already made with ingredients that are paleo-friendly.

Others can be made to be paleo by making some adjustments.

For example, if there is not something on the menu that you think is paleo, you can always order a salad with grilled chicken or fish.

As you transition into the paleo diet, it is normal to have some withdrawal symptoms.

These only last a few days for most people.

During this time, drink lots of water and get plenty of sleep.

It can also be helpful to make changes slowly instead of all at once, so it becomes a habit more easily.

Have a nice diet !!

Recipes

Breakfast

1.1 - Turkey Stuffed Mushroom Caps

Preparation time: 5 minutes
Cooking time: 10 minutes
Servings: **1**

Ingredients:

- 2 Portobello mushroom caps
- 2 lettuce leaves
- 2 avocado slices
- ½ pound turkey meat, cooked, sliced
- Olive oil

Directions:

1. Heat up a pan over medium-high heat, add the turkey meat, cook for 4 minutes, transfer to paper towels to drain excess oil.
2. Heat up the pan with the olive oil over medium high heat, add mushroom caps, cook for 2 minutes on each side and take off heat.
3. Arrange 1 mushroom cap on a plate, add turkey, avocado slices, and lettuce leaves, top with the other mushroom cap and serve.

Nutritional Values (Per Serving):

Calories: 521

Carbs: 3,1 g
Fat: 25,5 g
Fiber: 0,9 g
Protein: 67,9 g

1.2 - Turkey and Beef Patties

Preparation time: 10 minutes
Cooking time: 20 minutes
Servings: **1**

Ingredients:

- 5 eggs
- 1 pound ground beef meat
- ½ cup turkey meat, minced
- 4 small shallots
- 3 sun-dried tomatoes, chopped
- 2 teaspoons basil leaves, chopped
- 1 teaspoon garlic, minced
- A drizzle of olive oil
- Black pepper to taste

Directions:

1. In a bowl, combine the meat with 1 egg, tomatoes, basil, black pepper and garlic, stir and shape 4 burgers.
2. Heat up a pan over medium-high heat, add the burgers, cook them 5 minutes on each side and transfer them to a plate.
3. Heat up the same pan over medium-high heat, place the turkey patties, cook for 20 minutes and transfer it to a plate as well.
4. Heat up the pan again, add the chopped shallots and extra olive oil, cook for 4 minutes, drain excess oil and add next to the turkey patties.

5. Fry the remaining eggs in a pan with a drizzle of oil over a medium-high heat and place them on top of the burgers.
6. Top with the turkey patties and shallots and serve for breakfast.

Nutritional Values (Per Serving):

Calories: 406

Carbs: 14,8 g
Fat: 18,1 g
Fiber: 1,1 g
Protein: 45,5 g

1.3 - Basil Pork and Mushroom Pan

Preparation time: 10 minutes
Cooking time: 20 minutes
Servings: **4**

Ingredients:

- 8 ounces mushrooms, chopped
- 1 pound pork, ground
- 1 tablespoon olive oil
- 2 zucchinis, cubed
- ½ teaspoon garlic powder
- ½ teaspoon basil, dried
- A pinch of sea salt and black pepper
- 2 tablespoons Dijon mustard

Directions:

1. Heat up a pan with the oil over medium-high heat, add mushrooms, stir and cook for 4 minutes.
2. Add zucchinis, salt and black pepper, stir and cook for 4 minutes more.
3. Add pork, garlic powder and basil, stir and cook for 10 minutes.
4. Add the mustard, stir well, cook for a 3 more minutes, divide between plates and serve.

Nutritional Values (Per Serving):

Calories: 226

Carbs: 5,8 g
Fat: 8,1 g
Fiber: 1,9 g
Protein: 33,1 g

1.4 - Shallot and Coconut Muffins

Preparation time: 10 minutes
Cooking time: 25 minutes
Servings: **12**

Ingredients:

- 6 small shallots, peeled, chopped
- 1 yellow onion, chopped
- 4 avocados, pitted, peeled and mashed
- 4 eggs
- ½ cup coconut flour
- 1 cup coconut milk
- ½ teaspoon baking soda
- A pinch of sea salt and black pepper

Directions:

1. Heat up a pan over medium-high heat, add the shallots and onion, stir and cook for 5 minutes.
2. In a bowl, mix the avocados with the eggs, salt, black pepper, milk, baking soda and coconut flour and stir.
3. Add the shallots and onions, stir well again and divide into muffin pans.
4. Place in the oven at 350 degrees F and bake for 20 minutes.
5. Divide the muffins between plates and serve.

Nutritional Values (Per Serving):

Calories: 252

Carbs: 15,6 g
Fat: 20,3 g
Fiber: 9,1 g
Protein: 5,2 g

1.5 - Stuffed Mushrooms

Preparation time: 10 minutes
Cooking time: 15 minutes
Servings: **3**

Ingredients:

- 3 Portobello mushroom caps
- 10 oz turkey meat, cooked, sliced
- 3 eggs
- 4 ounces smoked salmon
- Olive oil

Directions:

1. Heat up a pan over medium-high heat, add the turkey, cook for 4 minutes, transfer to paper towels to drain excess oil.
2. Heat up the pan with the olive oil over medium heat, place egg rings in the pan, crack an egg in each, cook them for 6 minutes and transfer them to a plate.
3. Heat up the pan again over medium-high heat, add mushroom caps, cook for 5 minutes and transfer them to a platter.
4. Top each mushroom cap with turkey slices, salmon, and eggs and serve.

Nutritional Values (Per Serving):

Calories: 315

Carbs: 1,8 g
Fat: 15,5 g
Fiber: 0,4 g
Protein: 40,8 g

1.6 - Hot Chicken and Coconut Waffles

Preparation time: 10 minutes
Cooking time: 10 minutes
Servings: **4**

Ingredients:

- 1 and ½ cups chicken meat, cooked and shredded ½ cup hot sauce
- 1 cup almond flour
- 2 green onions, chopped
- ½ cup tapioca flour
- 2 eggs
- 6 tablespoon coconut flour
- ¾ teaspoons baking soda
- 1 teaspoon garlic powder
- 1 cup coconut milk
- ¼ cup ghee, melted
- Cooking spray
- A pinch of sea salt

Directions:

1. In a bowl, mix all the ingredients except the cooking spray and whisk well.
2. Pour some of the batter into your waffle iron greased with cooking spray, close the lid and make your waffle.
3. Repeat with the rest of the batter, divide waffles between plates and serve.

Nutritional Values (Per Serving):

Calories: 220

Carbs: 7 g
Fat: 15 g
Fiber: 1 g
Protein: 7 g

1.7 - Smoked Turkey Meatballs

Preparation time: 10 minutes
Cooking time: 20 minutes
Servings: **8**

Ingredients:

- 2 eggs
- 1 teaspoon baking soda
- 1 pound turkey meat, ground
- ¼ cup coconut flour
- Black pepper to taste
- 1 teaspoon smoked paprika

Directions:

1. In a food processor, mix the turkey meat with eggs, baking soda, flour, pepper and paprika, pulse well and shape medium balls out of this mix.
2. Arrange them on a lined baking sheet, bake them in the oven at 350 degrees F for 35 minutes, divide between plates and serve.

Nutritional Values (Per Serving):

Calories: 166

Carbs: 5,2 g
Fat: 7,5 g
Fiber: 5,5 g
Protein: 19,8 g

1.8 - Almond Berry Bowls

Preparation time: 5 minutes
Cooking time: 0 minutes
Servings: **2**

Ingredients:

- 2 tablespoons pumpkin seeds
- 2 tablespoons almonds, chopped
- 1 tablespoon chia seeds
- A handful blueberries
- 1 cup almond milk

Directions:

1. Divide the almond milk into 2 bowls, then divide the seeds, almonds and blueberries, toss to combine and serve.

Nutritional Values (Per Serving):

Calories: 400

Carbs: 16,4 g
Fat: 37,1 g
Fiber: 6,2 g
Protein: 7,2 g

1.9 - Ground Meat and Onion Pan

Preparation time: 10 minutes
Cooking time: 35 minutes
Servings: **8**

Ingredients:

- 1 pound pork meat, ground
- 1 pound turkey meat, ground
- A pinch of sea salt and black pepper
- 8 eggs, whisked
- 3 tablespoons ghee, melted
- 1 avocado, pitted, peeled and chopped
- 1 tomato, chopped
- ½ cup red onion, chopped
- 2 tablespoons tomato sauce

Directions:

---

1. In a bowl, mix the pork with turkey, salt and black pepper and combine.
2. Spread this on a lined baking sheet, shape a circle, spread the tomato sauce all over and bake at 350 degrees F for 25 minutes.
3. Heat up a pan with the ghee over medium heat, add the eggs, stir and scramble them for 5 minutes
4. Spread this over the pork mix, add the onion, tomato, and avocado, divide between plates and serve.

Nutritional Values (Per Serving):

Calories: 456

Carbs: 5 g
Fat: 35 g
Fiber: 2 g
Protein: 29,9 g

1.10 - Coconut Smoothie

Preparation time: 5 minutes
Cooking time: 0 minutes
Servings: **2**

Ingredients:

- 1 cup ice
- 2 peaches, peeled and chopped
- 1 teaspoon lemon zest, grated
- 1 cup cold coconut milk

Directions:

1. In a blender, combine all the ingredients and pulse well. Divide into glasses and serve.

Nutritional Values (Per Serving):

Calories: 336

Carbs: 20,9 g
Fat: 29 g
Fiber: 5 g
Protein: 4,2 g

Soups and Stews

2.1 - Cilantro Beef Stew

Preparation time: 10 minutes
Cooking time: 2 hours and 30 minutes
Servings: **4**

Ingredients:

- 2 pounds beef meat, cubed
- 3 yellow onions, chopped
- Black pepper to taste
- 2 tablespoons Moroccan spices
- 1/3 cup ghee, melted
- 2 cups beef stock
- 3 garlic cloves, minced
- 1 lemon, sliced
- Juice of 1 lemon
- Zest from 1 lemon, grated
- 1 butternut squash, peeled, seeded and cubed
- 1 bunch cilantro, chopped

Directions:

1. Heat up a Dutch oven with the ghee over medium heat, add beef, onions, spices, black pepper, garlic, lemon slices, lemon juice and zest and stock, toss and bake at 300 degrees F for 2 hours.
2. Add cilantro and squash, stir, bake for 30 minutes more, divide into bowls and serve.

Nutritional Values (Per Serving):

Calories: 627

Carbs: 14 g
Fat: 33,5 g
Fiber: 2,9 g
Protein: 65 g

2.2 - Pumpkin and Chicken Stew

Preparation time: 15 minutes
Cooking time: 8 hours
Servings: **6**

Ingredients:

- 5 garlic cloves, minced
- 2 celery stalks, chopped
- 2 yellow onions, chopped
- 2 carrots, chopped
- 30 ounces homemade pumpkin puree
- 2 quarts chicken stock
- 2 cups chicken breast, skinless, boneless and cubed
- ¼ cup coconut flour
- Black pepper to taste
- ½ pound baby spinach
- ¼ teaspoon cayenne pepper

Directions:

1. In a slow cooker, combine all the ingredients except the spinach, cover and cook on Low for 7 hours and 50 minutes.
2. Add the spinach, cook on Low for 10 more minutes, divide into bowls and serve.

Nutritional Values (Per Serving):

Calories: 222

Carbs: 30 g
Fat: 3,6 g
Fiber: 10,8 g
Protein: 18,6 g

2.3 - Cayenne Tomato and Eggplant Stew

Preparation time: 10 minutes
Cooking time: 30 minutes
Servings: **3**

Ingredients:

- 1 eggplant, chopped
- 1 yellow onion, chopped
- 2 tomatoes, chopped
- 1 teaspoon cumin powder
- A pinch of sea salt and black pepper
- 1 cup tomato puree
- A pinch of cayenne pepper
- ½ cup water

Directions:

1. Heat up a saucepan over medium-high heat, add the water, tomato paste, salt, pepper, cayenne and cumin and stir well.
2. Add the eggplant, tomato, and onion, stir, bring to a boil, reduce heat to medium, cook for 30 minutes, divide into bowls and serve.

Nutritional Values (Per Serving):

Calories: 102

Carbs: 23,4 g
Fat: 0,8 g
Fiber: 8,8 g
Protein: 4,1 g

2.4 - Coconut Sprouts Cream

Preparation time: 10 minutes
Cooking time: 20 minutes
Servings: **4**

Ingredients:

- 2 tablespoons olive oil
- 1 yellow onion, chopped
- 2 pounds Brussels sprouts, trimmed and halved
- 4 cups chicken stock
- ¼ cup coconut cream
- A pinch of black pepper

Directions:

1. Heat up a large saucepan with the oil over medium high heat, add the onion, stir and cook for 3 minutes.
2. Add Brussels sprouts, stir and cook for 2 minutes.
3. Add stock and black pepper, stir, bring to a simmer and cook for 20 minutes.
4. Blend using an immersion blender, add coconut cream, stir well, ladle into bowls and serve right away and serve.

Nutritional Values (Per Serving):

Calories: 153

Carbs: 24,8 g
Fat: 4,9 g
Fiber: 9,4 g
Protein: 9,1 g

2.5 - Mushrooms and Kale Soup

Preparation time: 10 minutes
Cooking time: 15 minutes
Servings: **4**

Ingredients:

- 1 yellow onion, chopped
- 2 carrots, chopped
- 6 mushrooms, chopped
- 1 red chili pepper, chopped
- 2 celery sticks, chopped
- 1 tablespoon coconut oil
- A pinch of sea salt and black pepper
- 4 garlic cloves, minced
- 4 ounces kale, chopped
- 15 oz fresh tomatoes, peeled, chopped
- 1 zucchini, chopped
- 1-quart veggie stock
- 1 bay leaf
- A handful parsley, chopped for serving

Directions:

1. Set your instant pot on Sauté mode, add oil and heat it up.
2. Add celery, carrots, onion, a pinch of salt and black pepper, stir and cook for 2 minutes.
3. Add chili pepper, garlic and the mushrooms, stir and cook for 2 minutes.
4. Add tomatoes, stock, bay leaf, kale and zucchinis, stir, cover pot and cook on High for 10 minutes.

5. Release pressure, stir soup again, discard the bay leaf, ladle into bowls, sprinkle the parsley on top and serve.

Nutritional Values (Per Serving):

Calories: 109

Carbs: 16,9 g
Fat: 3,9 g
Fiber: 4,3 g
Protein: 4,1 g

2.6 - Baharat Stew

Preparation time: 10 minutes
Cooking time: 8 hours
Servings: **6**

Ingredients:

- 1 cup carrots, chopped
- 1 cup celery, chopped
- 2 cups onions, chopped
- 3 pounds osso buco, bones in
- 4 garlic cloves, minced
- 6 teaspoons baharat
- A pinch of black pepper
- 2 cups beef stock
- A handful parsley, chopped
- 1 kale, chopped

Directions:

1. In a slow cooker, combine all the ingredients except the kale and the parsley, toss, cover and cook on Low for 7 hours and 30 minutes.
2. Add the kale, cook the stew on Low for 30 minutes more, divide into bowls, sprinkle the parsley on top and serve.

Nutritional Values (Per Serving):

Calories: 291

Carbs: 7,1 g
Fat: 7,9 g
Fiber: 1,7 g
Protein: 42,8 g

Preparation time: 10 minutes
Cooking time: 8 hours
Servings: **4**

Ingredients:

- 2 and ½ pounds beef chuck, cubed
- 3 cups collard greens
- 3 cups water
- 3 tablespoons allspice
- ¼ cup garlic powder
- 1/3 cup sweet paprika
- 1 teaspoon cayenne pepper
- 1 teaspoon chili powder

Directions:

1. In a slow cooker, combine all the ingredients, toss, cover and cook on Low for 8 hours.
2. Divide into bowls and serve.

Nutritional Values (Per Serving):

Calories: 953

Carbs: 15,9 g
Fat: 67,3 g
Fiber: 6,1 g
Protein: 71,4 g

2.8 - Coconut Cauliflower and Clam Cream

Preparation time: 10 minutes
Cooking time: 30 minutes
Servings: **6**

Ingredients:

- 1 small cauliflower head, florets separated
- 2 tablespoons coconut oil, melted
- 2 cups chicken stock
- 2 carrots, chopped
- 1 yellow onion, chopped
- 2 sweet potatoes, chopped
- 17 ounces cooked fresh clams
- 1 celery rib, chopped
- 1 cup coconut milk
- A pinch of sea salt and black pepper

Directions:

1. Heat up a large saucepan with half of the oil over medium-high heat, add half of the onion, cauliflower, and stock, stir, bring to a boil and cook for 10 minutes.
2. Blend with an immersion blender, and transfer this to a bowl.
3. Heat up the same saucepan with the rest of the oil over medium heat, add the rest of the onion, celery, carrot, salt and black pepper, stir and cook for 10 minutes.
4. Add potato, 2 cups of the cauliflower cream, stir, bring to a boil and simmer for 10 minutes.

5. Add coconut milk, clams and the rest of the cauliflower cream, stir, cook for 2 minutes more, ladle into soup bowls and serve.

Nutritional Values (Per Serving):

Calories: 260

Carbs: 31,6 g
Fat: 14,6 g
Fiber: 5,4 g
Protein: 3,7 g

2.9 - Coconut Zucchini Cream

Preparation time: 10 minutes
Cooking time: 20 minutes
Servings: **4**

Ingredients:

- 1 onion, chopped
- 3 zucchinis, cut into medium chunks
- 2 tablespoons coconut milk
- 2 garlic cloves, minced
- 4 cups chicken stock
- 2 tablespoons coconut oil
- A pinch of sea salt and black pepper

Directions:

1. Heat up a large saucepan with the oil over medium heat, add zucchinis, garlic, and onion, stir and cook for 5 minutes.
2. Add stock, salt, pepper, stir, bring to a boil, cover pan, simmer soup for 20 minutes and take off heat.
3. Add coconut milk, blend using an immersion blender, ladle into bowls and serve.

Nutritional Values (Per Serving):

Calories: 122

Carbs: 9,1 g
Fat: 9,5 g
Fiber: 2,4 g
Protein: 3 g

2.10 - Lemon Asparagus and Zucchini Cream

Preparation time: 10 minutes
Cooking time: 25 minutes
Servings: **3**

Ingredients:

- 1 celery stick, chopped
- 1 zucchini, chopped
- 1 yellow onion, chopped
- 2 pounds asparagus, trimmed and roughly chopped
- 2 garlic cloves, minced
- Grated lemon peel from ½ lemon
- Black pepper to taste
- 2 cups water
- 1 tablespoon olive oil

Directions:

1. Put the asparagus, zucchini, celery, onion, lemon peel and garlic on a lined baking sheet, drizzle the oil, season with black pepper, place in the oven at 400 degrees F and bake for 25 minutes.
2. Transfer these to a food processor, add the water and pulse well.
3. Transfer soup to a saucepan, heat up over medium heat for 1-2 minutes, ladle into bowls and serve right away.

Nutritional Values (Per Serving):

Calories: 132

Carbs: 18,6 g
Fat: 5,2 g
Fiber: 8,2 g
Protein: 8,1 g

Side Dishes

3.1 - Spinach and Pumpkin Mix

Preparation time: 10 minutes
Cooking time: 30 minutes
Servings: **6**

Ingredients:

- 2 tablespoons olive oil + 2 teaspoons olive oil
- 21 ounces pumpkin, peeled, seeded and cubed
- 2 teaspoons sesame seeds
- 1 tablespoon lemon juice
- 2 teaspoons mustard
- 4 ounces baby spinach
- 2 tablespoons pine nuts, toasted
- A pinch of sea salt and black pepper

Directions:

1. In a bowl, mix pumpkin with salt, black pepper and 2 teaspoons oil, toss to coat well, spread on a lined baking sheet, place in the oven at 400 degrees F and bake for 25 minutes.
2. Leave pumpkin pieces to cool down a bit, add sesame seeds, toss to coat, place in the oven again and bake for 5 minutes more.
3. In a bowl, mix lemon juice with the rest of the oil and mustard and whisk.
4. Leave pumpkin to completely cool down and transfer it to a salad bowl.
5. Add baby spinach, pine nuts and the salad dressing, toss to coat well, divide between plates and serve as a side salad.

Calories: 149

Carbs: 9,8 g
Fat: 12,5 g
Fiber: 3,7 g
Protein: 2,5 g

3.2 - Lemon Broccoli

Preparation time: 10 minutes
Cooking time: 20 minutes
Servings: **4**

Ingredients:

- 1 and ½ pounds broccoli
- 2 tablespoons lemon juice
- A pinch of sea salt
- 3 tablespoons avocado oil

Directions:

1. In a bowl, mix broccoli with a pinch of salt, oil and lemon juice, toss to coat well, spread on a lined baking sheet, place in the oven at 450 degrees F and roast for 20 minutes.
2. Divide them between plates and serve.

Nutritional Values (Per Serving):

Calories: 76

Carbs: 12,7 g
Fat: 1,9 g
Fiber: 5,2 g
Protein: 5,2 g

3.3 - Artichoke and Shallots Mix

Preparation time: 10 minutes
Cooking time: 1 hour and 10 minutes
Servings: **4**

Ingredients:

- 4 artichokes, stems cut off and hearts chopped
- 3 garlic cloves, minced
- 2 cups spinach, chopped
- 1 tablespoon coconut oil, melted
- 1 yellow onion, chopped
- 4 ounces shallots, chopped, cooked and crumbled A pinch of black pepper

Directions:

1. Put artichokes in a large saucepan, add water to cover, bring to a boil over medium heat, cook for 30 minutes, drain them and leave them aside to cool down.
2. Heat up a pan with the oil over medium high heat, add onion, stir and cook for 10 minutes.
3. Add spinach, stir, cook for 3 minutes, take off heat and leave aside to cool down.
4. Put cooked shallots in your food processor, add artichoke insides as well and pulse well.
5. Add this to spinach and onion mix and stir well.
6. Place artichoke cups on a lined baking sheet, stuff them with spinach mix, place in the oven at 375 degrees F and bake for 30 minutes.
7. Divide the artichokes between plates and serve as a side dish.

Nutritional Values (Per Serving):

Calories: 144

Carbs: 25,6 g
Fat: 3,8 g
Fiber: 9,7 g
Protein: 6,9 g

3.4 - Apple and Squash Mix

Preparation time: 10 minutes
Cooking time: 30 minutes
Servings: **4**

Ingredients:

- ½ teaspoon cinnamon powder
- 2 tablespoons olive oil
- 2 apples, peeled, cored and cubed
- 1 and ½ pounds butternut squash, peeled, seeded and cubed

Directions:

1. In a baking dish, toss well to combine all ingredients, place in the oven at 350 degrees F and roast for 30 minutes.
2. Divide between plates and serving.

Nutritional Values (Per Serving):

Calories: 221

Carbs: 42,3 g
Fat: 7,5 g
Fiber: 11 g
Protein: 2,6 g

3.5 - Cauliflower and Artichokes

Preparation time: 10 minutes
Cooking time: 20 minutes
Servings: **4**

Ingredients:

- 1 and ½ cups leeks, chopped
- 1 and ½ cups cauliflower florets
- 2 garlic cloves, minced
- 1 and ½ cups artichoke hearts
- 2 tablespoons coconut oil, melted
- Black pepper to taste

Directions:

1. Heat up a pan with the oil over medium-high heat, add garlic, leeks, cauliflower florets and artichoke hearts, stir and cook for 20 minutes.
2. Add black pepper, stir, divide between plates and serve.

Nutritional Values (Per Serving):

Calories: 192

Carbs: 35,1 g
Fat: 6,9 g
Fiber: 8,2 g
Protein: 5,1 g

3.6 - Fried Tapioca Root

Preparation time: 10 minutes
Cooking time: 1 hour
Servings: **4**

Ingredients:

- 2 and ½ pound tapioca root, cut in medium fries
- ½ cup ghee, melted
- Black pepper to taste

Directions:

1. Put some water in a large saucepan, bring to a boil over medium high heat, add tapioca fries, boil for 10 minutes and drain them well.
2. Spread the fries on a lined baking sheet, add black pepper and the ghee, toss everything to coat well, place in the oven at 375 degrees F and bake for 45 minutes.
3. Divide them between plates and serve as a side.

Nutritional Values (Per Serving):

Calories: 905

Carbs: 168,5 g
Fat: 25,5 g
Fiber: 1,7 g
Protein: 0,4 g

3.7 - Sage Squash Mix

Preparation time: 10 minutes
Cooking time: 55 minutes
Servings: **4**

Ingredients:

- 1 spaghetti squash, cut in halves and seeded
- 12 sage leaves, chopped
- 3 tablespoons ghee, melted
- A pinch of sea salt
- Black pepper to taste

Directions:

1. Place spaghetti squash on a lined baking sheet, place in the oven at 375 degrees F, bake for 40 minutes, and scoop strings of flesh into a bowl.
2. Heat up a pan with the ghee over medium heat, add sage, cook for 5 minutes and transfer them to paper towels.
3. Heat up the pan again over medium heat, add spaghetti squash, salt and black pepper to the taste, stir and cook for 3 minutes.
4. Add the sage, stir, divide between plates and serve as a side.

Nutritional Values (Per Serving):

Calories: 108

Carbs: 4,8 g
Fat: 10,3 g
Fiber: 2 g
Protein: 0,7 g

3.8 - Dill Zucchini Pan

Preparation time: 10 minutes
Cooking time: 7 minutes
Servings: **4**

Ingredients:

- 2 tablespoons mint
- 2 zucchinis, halved lengthwise and then slice into half moons
- 1 tablespoon coconut oil, melted
- ½ tablespoon dill, chopped
- A pinch of cayenne pepper

Directions:

1. Heat up a pan with the oil over medium-high heat, add zucchinis, stir and cook for 6 minutes.
2. Add cayenne, dill and mint, stir, cook for 1 minute more, divide between plates and serve.

Nutritional Values (Per Serving):

Calories: 46

Carbs: 3,5 g
Fat: 3,6 g
Fiber: 1,3 g
Protein: 1,3 g

3.9 - Turnip and Mushroom Mix

Preparation time: 10 minutes
Cooking time: 15 minutes
Servings: **4**

Ingredients:

- 1 teaspoon ginger, grated
- 1 pound white mushrooms, sliced
- 1 bunch turnip greens, trimmed
- 2 garlic cloves, minced
- Black pepper to taste
- A pinch of sea salt
- ½ cup raw almonds, chopped
- ¼ cup lime juice
- 2 tablespoons coconut oil, melted
- 1 tablespoon coconut aminos

Directions: .

1. Heat up a pan with the oil over medium high heat, add mushrooms and turnips greens, stir and cook for 2 minutes.
2. Add ginger and garlic, stir and cook for 2 minutes more.
3. Add lime juice, almonds, coconut aminos, salt and black pepper, stir and cook for 10 minutes more.
4. Divide between plates and serve.

Nutritional Values (Per Serving):

Calories: 164

Carbs: 9,4 g
Fat: 13,2 g
Fiber: 3,2 g
Protein: 6,5 g

3.10 - Pomegranate and Sprouts Mix

Preparation time: 10 minutes
Cooking time: 30 minutes
Servings: **6**

Ingredients:

- 1 and ½ pounds Brussels sprouts, halved A pinch of sea salt and black pepper
- 1 teaspoon garlic powder
- 2/3 cups pecans, chopped
- 1 cup pomegranate seeds
- 2 tablespoons extra virgin olive oil

Directions:

1. In a baking dish, combine all the ingredients except the pomegranate seeds, toss and bake at 400 degrees F for 30 minutes.
2. Divide between plates, top with pomegranate seeds and serve as a side dish.

Nutritional Values (Per Serving):

Calories: 184

Carbs: 15,3 g
Fat: 13,4 g
Fiber: 5,3 g
Protein: 5 g

Snacks and Appetizers

4.1 - Tahini Cauliflower Spread

Preparation time: 10 minutes
Cooking time: 45 minutes
Servings: **6**

Ingredients:

- 1 cauliflower head, florets separated
- ½ cup sun-dried tomatoes, chopped
- 10 garlic cloves
- 4 tablespoons tahini
- 4 tablespoons lemon juice
- 5 tablespoons olive oil
- 1 teaspoon basil, dried
- Black pepper to taste
- 1 teaspoon cumin, ground
- A pinch of sea salt

Directions:

1. Put cauliflower florets and garlic cloves on a lined baking sheet, drizzle 1 tablespoon oil over them, toss to coat, place in the oven at 400 degrees F and bake for 45 minutes flipping once.
2. Leave cauliflower and garlic to cool down and transfer to a blender.
3. Add sun-dried tomatoes, 4 tablespoons oil, black pepper, ½ teaspoon cumin, tahini paste, a pinch of salt and lemon juice and blend until you obtain a paste.
4. Transfer to a bowl, sprinkle the rest of the cumin and dried basil on top and serve.

Nutritional Values (Per Serving):

Calories: 183

Carbs: 6,9 g
Fat: 17,2 g
Fiber: 2,4 g
Protein: 3,1 g

4.2 - Zucchini Wraps

Preparation time: 10 minutes
Cooking time: 5 minutes
Servings: **4**

Ingredients:

- 3 zucchinis, thinly sliced lengthwise
- 10 ounces turkey meat, cooked, sliced into thin strips ½ cup sun-dried tomatoes, drained and chopped
- 4 tablespoons raspberry vinegar
- ½ cup basil, chopped
- A pinch of sea salt
- Black pepper to taste

Directions:

1. Place zucchini slices in a bowl, sprinkle a pinch of sea salt and vinegar over them and leave aside for 10 minutes.
2. Drain well and season with black pepper to taste.
3. Divide turkey slices, chopped sun dried tomatoes and basil over zucchini ones, roll each and secure with a toothpick and arrange them on a lined baking sheet.
4. Place in the oven at 400 degrees F for 5 minutes, then arrange them on a platter and serve as an appetizer.

Nutritional Values (Per Serving):

Calories: 152

Carbs: 6 g
Fat: 3,9 g
Fiber: 1,9 g
Protein: 22,8 g

4.3 - Cheese Bites

Preparation time: 5 minutes
Cooking time: 10 minutes
Servings: **24 pieces**

Ingredients:

- 1/3 cup tomatoes, chopped
- ½ cup bell peppers, mixed and chopped
- ½ cup tomato sauce
- 4 ounces almond cheese, cubed
- 2 tablespoons basil, chopped
- Black pepper to taste

Directions:

1. Divide tomato and bell pepper pieces into a muffin tray.
2. Also divide the tomato sauce, basil and almond cheese cubes, sprinkle black pepper at the end, place cups in the oven at 400 degrees F and bake for 10 minutes.
3. Arrange the meal on a platter and serve.

Nutritional Values (Per Serving):

Calories: 59

Carbs: 2 g
Fat: 4,5 g
Fiber: 0,1 g
Protein: 2,5 g

4.4 - Squash Wraps

Preparation time: 10 minutes
Cooking time: 40 minutes
Servings: **4**

Ingredients:

- 10 ounces turkey meat, cooked, sliced
- 2 pounds butternut squash, cubed
- 1 teaspoon chili powder
- 1 teaspoon garlic powder
- 1 teaspoon sweet paprika
- Black pepper to taste

Directions:

1. In a bowl, mix butternut squash cubes with chili powder, black pepper, garlic powder and paprika and toss to coat.
2. Wrap squash pieces in turkey slices, place them all on a lined baking sheet, place in the oven at 350 degrees F, bake for 20 minutes, flip and bake for 20 minutes more.
3. Arrange squash bites on a platter and serve.

Nutritional Values (Per Serving):

Calories: 223

Carbs: 26,5 g
Fat: 3,8 g
Fiber: 4,5 g
Protein: 23 g

4.5 - Chives Cauliflower Bites

Preparation time: 5 minutes
Cooking time: 30 minutes
Servings: **1**

Ingredients:

- 1 small cauliflower head, chopped
- A pinch of sea salt
- ½ teaspoon chives, dried
- ½ teaspoon onion powder
- A drizzle of avocado oil

Directions:

1. In a bowl, mix cauliflower popcorn with a pinch of salt and the oil, toss to coat, spread them on a lined baking sheet, and bake at 450 degrees F for 30 minutes, tossing the popcorn halfway.
2. Transfer the popcorn to a bowl, add chives and onion powder, stir and serve them.

Nutritional Values (Per Serving):

Calories: 194

Carbs: 15 g
Fat: 14,3 g
Fiber: 6,7 g
Protein: 5,4 g

4.6 - Lemon Cashew Spread

Preparation time: 10 minutes
Cooking time: 0 minutes
Servings: **6**

Ingredients:

- ½ cup cashews, soaked for 2 hours and drained 1 tablespoon olive oil
- 2 tablespoons lemon juice
- ½ cup pumpkin puree
- 2 tablespoons sesame paste
- 1 garlic clove, minced
- ¼ teaspoon cumin, ground
- A pinch of cayenne pepper
- A pinch of sea salt
- ½ teaspoon pumpkin spice

Directions:

---

1. In your food processor, mix soaked cashews with lemon juice, pumpkin puree, sesame paste, garlic, cumin, pepper, sea salt and pumpkin spice and blend well.
2. Add oil gradually, blend again well, transfer to a bowl and serve as a snack.

Nutritional Values (Per Serving):

Calories: 99

Carbs: 5,7 g
Fat: 8,2 g
Fiber: 1 g
Protein: 2,2 g

Meat

5.1 - Beef and Mushrooms

Preparation time: 10 minutes
Cooking time: 3 hours
Servings: **4**

Ingredients:

- 1 yellow onion, sliced
- 3 garlic cloves, minced
- 1 cup beef stock
- 2 tablespoons coconut oil, melted
- 3 pounds beef, cubed
- A pinch of sea salt and black pepper
- 8 ounces carrots, sliced
- 8 ounces mushrooms, sliced
- 1 teaspoon thyme, chopped

Directions:

1. Heat up a Dutch oven with half of the oil over medium-high heat, add beef cubes, season with salt and black pepper, brown for 2 minutes on each side and transfer to a bowl.
2. Heat up the same Dutch oven over medium heat, add garlic, stir and cook for 2 minutes.
3. Add stock, stir well and heat it up.
4. Return meat to the pot, stir, place in the oven at 250 degrees F and roast for 3 hours.
5. In a bowl, mix carrots with mushrooms, the rest of the oil, salt, black pepper and thyme, stir well, spread these into a pan, place in the oven at 250 degrees F and roast them for 15 minutes.

6. Divide beef and juices between plates and serve with roasted veggies on the side.

Nutritional Values (Per Serving):

Calories: 745

Carbs: 10,9 g
Fat: 28,4 g
Fiber: 2,7 g
Protein: 106,6 g

5.2 - Parsley Lamb Mix

Preparation time: 10 minutes
Cooking time: 7 minutes
Servings: **4**

Ingredients:

- 8 lamb chops
- 2 tablespoons ras el hanout
- 1 teaspoon olive oil
- For the sauce:
- ¼ cup parsley, chopped
- 2 tablespoons mint, chopped
- 3 garlic cloves, minced
- 2 tablespoons lemon zest
- ¼ cup olive oil
- ½ teaspoon smoked paprika
- 1 teaspoon red pepper flakes
- 2 tablespoons lemon juice
- A pinch of sea salt
- Black pepper to taste

Directions:

1. Rub lamb chops with ras el hanout and 1 teaspoon oil, put them on preheated grill over medium-high heat, cook for 2 minutes on each side and divide them between plates.
2. In a food processor, mix parsley with mint, garlic, lemon zest, ¼ cup oil, paprika, pepper flakes, lemon juice, a pinch of salt and black pepper and pulse really well.
3. Drizzle this over lamb chops and serve.

Nutritional Values (Per Serving):

Calories: 551

Carbs: 2,4 g
Fat: 32,6 g
Fiber: 0,8 g
Protein: 60,2 g

5.3 - Broiled Lamb

Preparation time: 10 minutes
Cooking time: 10 minutes
Servings: **4**

Ingredients:

- 4 lamb chops
- 12 rosemary springs
- 4 garlic cloves, halved
- ½ teaspoon black peppercorns
- 3 tablespoons avocado oil
- A pinch of sea salt

Directions:

1. In a bowl, mix lamb chops with salt, black peppercorns and oil, rub well, place the chops in a lined baking sheet and add the garlic halves on top.
2. Rub rosemary into your palms and add over lamb chops.
3. Introduce everything in preheated broiler over medium-high heat for 10 minutes, divide between plates and serve.

Nutritional Values (Per Serving):

Calories: 634

Carbs: 2,8 g
Fat: 25,6 g
Fiber: 1,3 g
Protein: 92,3 g

5.4 - Chicken Balls and Sauce

Preparation time: 10 minutes
Cooking time: 20 minutes
Servings: **4**

Ingredients:

- 1 teaspoon sweet paprika
- 1 pineapple, diced
- 1 egg, whisked
- 2 pounds chicken meat, ground
- A pinch of sea salt
- Black pepper to taste
- 1 teaspoon garlic powder
- 1 teaspoon onion powder
- For the sauce:
- ¼ cup coconut amino
- 4 tablespoon paleo ketchup
- 1 tablespoon ginger, grated
- ½ cup pineapple juice
- 2 teaspoons raw honey
- ½ teaspoon red pepper flakes
- Salt and black pepper to taste
- 1 tablespoon garlic, minced

1. In a large saucepan, mix amino with ketchup, ginger, pineapple juice, garlic, pepper flakes, honey, a pinch of sea salt and pepper, stir well, bring to a boil over medium heat, simmer for 8 minutes and take off the heat.
2. In a bowl, mix chicken meat with paprika, egg, onion powder, garlic powder, salt and black pepper to taste and stir well.
3. Shape meatballs, arrange them on a lined baking sheet, place them in the oven at 475 degrees F and bake for 15 minutes.
4. Heat up a pan over medium heat, add pineapple pieces, stir and cook for 2 minutes.
5. Add baked meatballs, pour sauce you've made all over, stir gently, cook for 5 minutes, divide between plates and serve.

Nutritional Values (Per Serving):

Calories: 552

Carbs: 1,8 g
Fat: 18,3 g
Fiber: 26,2 g
Protein: 68,2 g

5.5 - Veal and Zucchini Wraps

Preparation time: 10 minutes
Cooking time: 20 minutes
Servings: **4**

Ingredients:

- 2 zucchinis, cut into quarters
- 8 veal scallops
- 2 tablespoons olive oil
- 2 teaspoons garlic powder
- ¼ cup balsamic vinegar
- A pinch of sea salt
- Black pepper to taste

Directions:

1. Flatten veal scallops with a meat tenderizer and season them with salt and black pepper.
2. Season zucchini salt, black pepper and garlic powder, place on preheated grill over medium-high heat, cook for 2 minutes on each side and transfer to a working surface.
3. Roll veal around each zucchini piece.
4. In a bowl, mix oil with balsamic vinegar and whisk well.
5. Brush veal rolls with this mix, place them on your grill and cook for 3 minutes on each side.
6. Serve right away.

Nutritional Values (Per Serving):

Calories: 136

Carbs: 5,9 g
Fat: 7,7 g
Fiber: 1,2 g
Protein: 11,5 g

5.6 - Orange Duck Mix

Preparation time: 10 minutes
Cooking time: 2 hours
Servings: **4**

Ingredients:

- 2 teaspoons allspice, ground
- 4 duck legs
- 4 thyme springs
- 1 lemon, sliced
- 1 orange, sliced
- 1 cup chicken broth
- A pinch of sea salt
- Black pepper to taste
- ½ cup orange juice

Directions:

1. Heat up a pan over medium-high heat, add duck legs, season with salt and pepper, and brown them for 3 minutes on each side.
2. Arrange half of lemon and orange slices on the bottom of a baking dish, place duck legs, top with the rest of the orange and lemon slices and thyme springs.
3. Add chicken stock, orange juice, sprinkle allspice, place in the oven at 350 degrees F and bake for 2 hours.
4. Divide between plates and serve hot.

Nutritional Values (Per Serving):

Calories: 187

Carbs: 2 g
Fat: 5,1 g
Fiber: 24 g
Protein: 11,3 g

5.7 - Cajun Steaks

Preparation time: 10 minutes
Cooking time: 25 minutes
Servings: **2**

Ingredients:

- 2 tablespoons Cajun spice
- ¼ cup coconut oil
- 2 medium skirt steaks
- 1/3 cup lemon juice
- ¼ cup apricot preserves
- ¼ cup coconut aminos

Directions:

1. In a bowl, mix half of the Cajun spice with lemon juice, aminos, oil and apricot preserves and stir well.
2. Pour this into a pan, bring to a boil over medium high heat and simmer for 8 minutes.
3. Blend this using an immersion blender and leave aside for now.
4. Season steaks with the rest of the Cajun spice, brush them with half of the apricots mix, place them on preheated grill over medium-high heat and cook them for 6-minute son each side.
5. Divide steaks on plates and top with the rest of the apricots mix.

Nutritional Values (Per Serving):

Calories: 887

Carbs: 31,1 g
Fat: 53,3 g
Fiber: 0,3 g
Protein: 68,7 g

5.8 - Coconut Beef Mix

Preparation time: 10 minutes
Cooking time: 20 minutes
Servings: **4**

Ingredients:

- 2 green onions, chopped
- 1 and ½ pounds steaks, sliced
- ¼ cup coconut sugar
- ½ cup coconut aminos
- 1 tablespoon ginger, minced
- 2 garlic cloves, minced
- ¼ cup pear juice
- 2 tablespoons olive oil

Directions:

1. Heat up a pan with half of the oil over medium heat, add ginger and garlic, stir and cook for 2 minutes.
2. Add the sugar, aminos, pear juice, stir, bring to a simmer and cook for 12 minutes.
3. Add tapioca mixed with the water, stir and cook until it thickens.
4. Heat up a pan with the rest of the oil over medium-high heat, add steak slices and brown them for 2 minutes on each side.
5. Add green onions and half of the sauce you've just made, stir gently and cook for 3 minutes more.
6. Divide steaks between plates and serve with the rest of the sauce on top.

Nutritional Values (Per Serving):

Calories: 487

Carbs: 17,6 g
Fat: 19,1 g
Fiber: 0,4 g
Protein: 58,5 g

5.9 - Cumin Lamb

Preparation time: 10 minutes
Cooking time: 2 hours and 30 minutes
Servings: **4**

Ingredients:

- 15 garlic cloves, peeled
- 2 teaspoons onion powder
- 6 lamb shanks
- 2 teaspoons cumin powder
- 1 cup water
- 3 teaspoons oregano, dried
- ½ cup olive oil
- A pinch of sea salt and black pepper
- ½ cup lemon juice

Directions:

1. In a roasting pan, combine all the ingredients, toss well and roast in the oven at 350 degrees F for 2 hours and 30 minutes.
2. Divide everything between plates and serve.

Nutritional Values (Per Serving):

Calories: 647

Carbs: 6,5 g
Fat: 41,4 g
Fiber: 1 g
Protein: 61,1 g

5.10 - Lamb and Squash Mix

Preparation time: 2 hours
Cooking time: 1 hour
Servings: **4**

Ingredients:

- 1 butternut squash, cubed
- 3 pounds lamb shoulder, chopped
- 4 shallots, chopped
- 4 carrots, chopped
- 4 tomatoes, chopped
- 2 Thai chilies, chopped
- 2 tablespoons tomato paste
- 1 cinnamon stick
- 2 and ½ cups warm beef broth
- 1 lemongrass stalk, finely chopped
- 1 teaspoon Chinese five spice powder
- 1 tablespoon ginger, minced
- 2 tablespoon coconut aminos
- 1 and ½ tablespoons coconut oil
- 3 garlic cloves, chopped
- Black pepper to taste

Directions:

1. In a bowl, mix lamb with coconut aminos, ginger, lemongrass, garlic and pepper, stir well, cover and keep in the fridge for 2 hours.
2. Heat up a pot with the oil over medium-high heat, add marinated lamb, stir and brown for 3 minutes.

3. Add tomato paste and tomatoes, stir and cook for 2 more minutes.
4. Add squash, shallots, Thai chilies, carrots, cinnamon stick, beef stock and five spices, stir well, place in the oven at 325 degrees F and bake for 1 hour.
5. Divide between plates and serve hot.

Nutritional Values (Per Serving):

Calories: 775

Carbs: 22,1 g
Fat: 29,6 g
Fiber: 33,9 g
Protein: 100,9 g

Fish and Seafood

Preparation time: 10 minutes
Cooking time: 20 minutes
Servings: **4**

Ingredients:

- 1 cup walnuts, chopped
- 4 salmon fillets, boneless
- ¼ cup lemon juice
- 2 tablespoons stevia
- 1 teaspoon dill, chopped
- A pinch of sea salt
- Black pepper to taste
- 1 tablespoon mustard

Directions:

1. In a bowl, mix the walnuts with mustard, stevia, lemon juice, a pinch of salt, black pepper and dill and stir well.
2. Spread this over salmon fillets, press well, place them on a lined baking sheet, place in the oven at 375 degrees F and bake for 20 minutes.
3. Divide salmon between plates and serve with a side salad.

Nutritional Values (Per Serving):

Calories: 446

Carbs: 4,5 g
Fat: 30,4 g
Fiber: 2,6 g
Protein: 42,9 g

Preparation time: 10 minutes
Cooking time: 12 minutes
Servings: **2**

Ingredients:

- 3 tablespoons ghee, melted
- 2 pound little clams, scrubbed
- 1 shallot, minced
- 2 garlic cloves, minced
- 1 cup cider
- 1 apple, cored and chopped
- Juice of ½ lemon

Directions:

1. Heat up a pan with the ghee over medium-high heat, add the shallot and garlic, stir and cook for 3 minutes.
2. Add cider, stir well and cook for 1 minute.
3. Add clams and thyme, cover and simmer for 5 minutes.
4. Add apple and lemon juice, stir, divide everything into bowls and serve.

Nutritional Values (Per Serving):

Calories: 610

Carbs: 43,7 g
Fat: 23,6 g
Fiber: 2,9 g
Protein: 55,1 g

6.3 - Maple Salmon

Preparation time: 10 minutes
Cooking time: 12 minutes
Servings: **4**

Ingredients:

- 2 tablespoons dill, chopped
- 4 salmon fillets, boneless
- 2 tablespoons chives, chopped
- 1/3 cup maple syrup
- A drizzle of olive oil
- 3 tablespoons balsamic vinegar
- A pinch of sea salt
- Black pepper to taste
- Lime wedges for serving

Directions:

1. Heat up a pan with the oil over medium-high heat, add fish fillets, season them with a pinch of sea salt and black pepper, cook for 3 minutes, cover pan and cook for 6 minutes more.
2. Add balsamic vinegar and maple syrup and cook for 3 minutes basting fish with this mix.
3. Add dill and chives, cook for 1 minute, divide the fish between plates and serve with lime wedges on the side.

Calories: 346

Carbs: 20,4 g
Fat: 14,7 g
Fiber: 0,7 g
Protein: 35 g

6.4 - Shrimp with Mushrooms

Preparation time: 10 minutes
Cooking time: 20 minutes
Servings: **4**

Ingredients:

- 1 tablespoon ghee, melted
- 1 cauliflower head, florets separated
- ¼ cup coconut milk
- 1 pound shrimp, peeled and deveined
- 2 garlic cloves, minced
- 8 ounces mushrooms, sliced
- 3 small shallots, peeled, sliced
- A pinch of red pepper flakes
- A handful mixed parsley and chives, chopped
- ½ cup beef stock
- Black pepper to taste

Directions:

1. Heat up a pan over medium-high heat, add shallots slices, cook for 3 minutes on each side, drain grease on paper towels and leave aside.
2. Put cauliflower florets in a food processor, blend until you obtain your "rice" and transfer to a heated pan over medium-high heat.
3. Cook cauliflower rice for 5 minutes stirring often.
4. Add coconut milk and 1 tablespoon ghee, stir and cook for a couple more minutes.

5. Blend everything using an immersion blender, add black pepper to taste, stir, reduce heat to low and cook for 3 more minutes
6. Heat up the pan where you cooked the shallots over medium-high heat, add the shrimp, cook for 2 minutes on each side and transfer to a plate.
7. Heat up the pan again over medium heat, add mushrooms, stir and cook for a few minutes.
8. Add garlic, pepper flakes and black pepper, stir and cook for 1 minute.
9. Add stock, return shrimp to pan, stir and cook for 4 minutes.
10. Divide cauliflower rice between plates, top with shrimp and mushrooms mix, top with crispy shallots and sprinkle parsley and chives on top.

Nutritional Values (Per Serving):

Calories: 241

Carbs: 10,7 g
Fat: 9,1 g
Fiber: 3,1 g
Protein: 30,4 g

6.5 - Parsley Scallops

Preparation time: 10 minutes
Cooking time: 0 minutes
Servings: **2**

Ingredients:

- Juice of ½ lemon
- 1 tablespoon green onions, chopped
- 1 tablespoon olive oil
- 6 scallops, chopped
- ½ tablespoons parsley, chopped
- A pinch of sea salt
- Black pepper to taste

Directions:

1. In a bowl, mix all the ingredients and stir well.
2. Divide into small cups and serve.

Nutritional Values (Per Serving):

Calories: 144

Carbs: 3,5 g
Fat: 7,7 g
Fiber: 0,2 g
Protein: 15,2 g

6.6 - Pesto Salmon Mix

Preparation time: 10 minutes
Cooking time: 15 minutes
Servings: **4**

Ingredients:

- 4 salmon fillets, skin on
- 1 tablespoon red bell pepper, chopped
- 1 shallot, chopped
- 2 tablespoon basil, chopped
- ½ cup cherry tomatoes, cut in quarters
- 2 garlic cloves, minced
- ½ cup sun-dried tomatoes, chopped
- 3 tablespoons olive oil
- A pinch of sea salt
- Black pepper to taste

Directions:

1. In a food processor, mix sun-dried tomatoes with garlic, oil, basil, shallots, a pinch of sea salt and black pepper and blend well.
2. Rub salmon with some of this mix, place under preheated broiler over medium-high heat, cook for 12 minutes flipping once and divide between plates.
3. Add the rest of the tomato pesto on top and serve with cherry tomatoes and bell pepper pieces on the side.

Nutritional Values (Per Serving):

Calories: 343

Carbs: 4,1 g
Fat: 21,6 g
Fiber: 0,7 g
Protein: 35,2 g

6.7 - Halibut and Peppers Slaw

Preparation time: 15 minutes
Cooking time: 10 minutes
Servings: **4**

Ingredients:

- 4 medium halibut fillets, skinless, boneless
- 2 teaspoons olive oil
- 4 teaspoons lemon juice
- 1 garlic clove, minced
- 1 teaspoon sweet paprika
- A pinch of sea salt
- Black pepper to taste
- For the salsa:
- ¼ cup green onions, chopped
- 1 cup red bell pepper, chopped
- 4 teaspoons oregano, chopped
- 1 small habanero pepper, chopped
- 1 garlic clove, minced
- ¼ cup lemon juice

Directions:

1. In a bowl, mix red bell pepper with habanero, green onion, ¼ cup lemon juice, 1 garlic clove, oregano, a pinch of sea salt and black pepper, stir well and keep in the fridge for now.
2. In a large bowl, mix paprika, olive oil, 1 garlic clove and 4 teaspoons lemon juice and stir well.
3. Add fish, rub well, cover bowl and leave aside for 10 minutes.

4. Place marinated fish under preheated broiler over medium-high heat, season with a pinch of sea salt and black pepper, cook for 4 minutes on each side and divide between plates.
5. Top fish with the salsa you've made earlier and serve.

Nutritional Values (Per Serving):

Calories: 402

Carbs: 0,6 g
Fat: 8,7 g
Fiber: 0,2 g
Protein: 75,7 g

6.8 - Salmon and Potato Mix

Preparation time: 10 minutes
Cooking time: 40 minutes
Servings: **2**

Ingredients:

- 2 salmon fillets, boneless
- 2 tablespoons mustard
- 1 tablespoon maple syrup
- A pinch of sea salt
- Black pepper to taste
- 2 sweet potatoes, peeled and chopped
- 2 teaspoons coconut oil
- ¼ cup coconut milk
- 3 garlic cloves, minced

Directions:

1. In a bowl, mix maple syrup with mustard and whisk well.
2. Season salmon fillets with a pinch of sea salt and black pepper to taste and brush them with half of the maple mix.
3. Heat up a pan with 1 teaspoon coconut oil over medium-high heat, add salmon, skin side down and cook for 4 minutes.
4. Transfer salmon to a baking dish, brush with the rest of the maple syrup mix, place in the oven at 425 degrees F and roast for 10 minutes.
5. Put sweet potatoes in a large saucepan, add water to cover, bring to a boil over medium heat, cover and cook for 20 minutes.

6. Heat up a pan with the rest of the oil over medium heat, add garlic, stir and cook for 1 minute.
7. Add sweet potatoes, stir well and then mash everything with a potato masher.
8. Add coconut milk, a pinch of salt and black pepper to taste and blend using an immersion blender.
9. Divide this mash between plates, add salmon on the side and serve.

Nutritional Values (Per Serving):

Calories: 606

Carbs: 55,6 g
Fat: 26,2 g
Fiber: 8,6 g
Protein: 40,6 g

6.9 - Scallops Salad

Preparation time: 10 minutes
Cooking time: 13 minutes
Servings: **4**

Ingredients:

- 1 shallot, minced
- 3 garlic cloves, minced
- 1 and ½ cups chicken stock
- ¼ cup walnuts, toasted and chopped
- 1 and ½ cups grapes, halved
- 2 cups spinach
- 1 tablespoon avocado oil
- 1 pound scallops
- A pinch of sea salt
- Black pepper to taste

Directions:

1. Heat up a pan with the oil over medium heat, add the shallot and the garlic, stir and cook for 2 minutes.
2. Add the walnuts, grapes, salt and pepper, stir and cook for 3 more minutes.
3. Add the scallops and cook them for 2 minutes on each side.
4. Add the spinach, toss, cook everything for 3 more minutes, divide everything into bowls and serve.

Nutritional Values (Per Serving):

Calories: 205

Carbs: 17,5 g
Fat: 7,4 g
Fiber: 1,5 g
Protein: 24,9 g

6.10 - Chili Salmon Mix

Preparation time: 20 minutes
Cooking time: 10 minutes
Servings: **4**

Ingredients:

- 1 teaspoon cumin, ground
- 1 teaspoon sweet paprika
- 1 teaspoon chili powder
- 1 teaspoon onion powder
- ½ teaspoon garlic powder
- 4 salmon fillets, boneless
- A pinch of sea salt
- Black pepper to taste
- For the avocado sauce:
- 2 avocados, pitted, peeled and chopped
- 1 garlic clove, minced
- Juice of 1 lime
- 1 red onion, chopped
- 1 tablespoon olive oil
- Black pepper to taste
- 1 tablespoon cilantro, finely chopped

Directions:

1. In a bowl, mix paprika with cumin, onion powder, garlic powder, chili powder, salt, pepper and the salmon, toss and keep in the fridge for 20 minutes.
2. Put avocado in a bowl, mash well with a fork, add red onion, garlic clove, lime juice, olive oil, chopped cilantro, and pepper to taste and stir.

3. Put the salmon on preheated grill over medium-high heat, cook for 3 minutes on each side and divide between plates.
4. Top each salmon piece with avocado sauce and serve.

Nutritional Values (Per Serving):

Calories: 494

Carbs: 14 g
Fat: 34,4 g
Fiber: 7,9 g
Protein: 37,2 g

Vegetables

7.1 - Peppers Pizza

Preparation time: 10 minutes
Cooking time: 30 minutes
Servings: **6**

Ingredients:

- 1 and ½ cups mashed cauliflower
- A pinch of sea salt
- Black pepper to taste
- ½ cup almond meal
- 1 and ½ tablespoons flax seed, ground
- 2/3 cup water
- ½ teaspoon oregano, dried
- ½ teaspoon garlic powder
- Tomato sauce for serving
- 2 tablespoons chives, chopped
- 2 tablespoons red bell peppers, chopped

Directions:

1. In a bowl, mix flax seed with water and stir well.
2. In a separate bowl, mix cauliflower with almond meal, flax seed mix, a pinch of sea salt, pepper, oregano and garlic powder, stir well, shape small pizza crusts, spread them on a lined baking sheet and bake them in the oven at 420 degrees F and bake for 15 minutes.
3. Take pizzas out of the oven, spread the tomato sauce all over, sprinkle the chives, and bell peppers, place in the oven again and bake 10 more minutes.
4. Divide between plates and serve.

Nutritional Values (Per Serving):

Calories: 145

Carbs: 11,2 g
Fat: 9,7 g
Fiber: 5,3 g
Protein: 5,5 g

7.2 - Hot Cucumber and Pepper Salad

Preparation time: 1 hour and 10 minutes
Cooking time: 0 minutes
Servings: **12**

Ingredients:

- 2 cucumbers, chopped
- ½ cup green bell pepper, chopped
- 2 tomatoes, chopped
- 1 jalapeno pepper, chopped
- 1 yellow onion, chopped
- 1 garlic clove, minced
- 2 teaspoons cilantro, chopped
- 1 teaspoon parsley, chopped
- 2 tablespoons lime juice
- ½ teaspoon dill weed
- A pinch of sea salt
- Black pepper to taste

Directions:

1. In a bowl, mix cucumbers with jalapeno, tomatoes, green pepper, garlic, onion, a pinch of sea salt and pepper to taste.
2. Add parsley, cilantro, dill and lime juice and stir well again.
3. Keep in the fridge for 1 hour and serve.

Nutritional Values (Per Serving):

Calories: 18

Carbs: 4,2 g
Fat: 0,1 g
Fiber: 0,8 g
Protein: 0,7 g

7.3 - Coconut Wraps

Preparation time: 40 minutes
Cooking time: 0 minutes
Servings: **4**

Ingredients:

- For the mayo:
- 1 tablespoon coconut aminos
- 3 tablespoons lemon juice
- 1 cup macadamia nuts
- 1 tablespoon maple syrup
- 1 teaspoon caraway seeds
- 1/3 cup dill, chopped
- A pinch of sea salt
- Some water
- For the filling:
- 1 cup alfalfa sprouts
- 1 red bell pepper, cut into thin strips
- 2 carrots, cut into thin matchsticks
- 1 cucumber, cut into thin matchsticks
- 1 cup pea shoots
- 4 Paleo coconut wrappers

Directions:

1. Put macadamia nuts in a bowl, add water to cover, leave aside for 30 minutes and drain well.
2. In a food processor, mix nuts with coconut aminos, lemon juice, maple syrup, caraway seeds, a pinch of salt and dill and blend very well.

3. Add some water and blend again until you obtain a smooth mayo.
4. Divide alfalfa sprouts, bell pepper, carrot, cucumber and pea shoots on each coconut wrappers, spread dill mayo over them, wrap, cut each in half and serve.

Nutritional Values (Per Serving):

Calories: 313

Carbs: 39,4 g
Fat: 26 g
Fiber: 6,4 g
Protein: 8,7 g

7.4 - Almond Eggplant Bake

Preparation time: 10 minutes
Cooking time: 30 minutes
Servings: **3**

Ingredients:

- 2 eggplants, sliced
- A pinch of sea salt
- Black pepper to taste
- 1 cup almonds, ground
- 1 teaspoon garlic, minced
- 2 teaspoons olive oil

Directions:

1. Grease a baking dish with some of the oil and arrange eggplant slices on it.
2. Season them with a pinch of salt and some black pepper and leave them aside for 10 minutes.
3. In a food processor, mix almonds with the rest of the oil, garlic, a pinch of salt and black pepper and blend well.
4. Spread this over eggplant slices, place in the oven at 425 degrees F and bake for 30 minutes.
5. Divide between plates and serve.

Nutritional Values (Per Serving):

Calories: 303

Carbs: 28,6 g
Fat: 19,6 g
Fiber: 16,9 g
Protein: 10,3 g

7.5 - Pesto Mushrooms

Preparation time: 10 minutes
Cooking time: 10 minutes
Servings: **4**

Ingredients:

- 12 big mushrooms, stems removed
- A pinch of sea salt
- Black pepper to taste
- 1 small tomato, diced
- ¼ cup homemade paleo pesto
- 2 tablespoons extra virgin olive oil

Directions:

1. Brush mushrooms with the olive oil and season them with a pinch of sea salt and pepper to taste.
2. Heat up a pan over medium-high heat, add mushrooms and cook them for 5 minutes on each side.
3. Transfer them to a platter, fill each with pesto sauce, top with diced tomatoes and serve.

Nutritional Values (Per Serving):

Calories: 134

Carbs: 3,7 g
Fat: 11,3 g
Fiber: 1 g
Protein: 6,9 g

7.6 - Zucchini Noodles Mix

Preparation time: 10 minutes
Cooking time: 20 minutes
Servings: **6**

Ingredients:

- 2 tablespoons olive oil
- 3 zucchinis, cut with a spiralizer
- 16 ounces mushrooms, sliced
- ¼ cup sun dried tomatoes, chopped
- 1 teaspoon garlic, minced
- ½ cup cherry tomatoes, halved
- 2 cups marinara sauce
- 2 cups spinach, chopped
- A pinch of sea salt
- Black pepper to taste
- A pinch of cayenne pepper
- A handful basil, chopped

Directions:

1. Put zucchini noodles in a bowl, season them with a pinch of salt and black pepper and leave them aside for 10 minutes.
2. Heat up a pan with the oil over medium-high heat, add garlic, stir and cook for 1 minute.
3. Add mushrooms, stir and cook for 4 minutes.
4. Add sun dried tomatoes, stir and cook for 4 minutes more.
5. Add cherry tomatoes, spinach, cayenne, marinara and zucchini noodles, stir and cook for 6 minutes more.

6. Sprinkle basil on top, toss gently, divide between plates and serve.

Nutritional Values (Per Serving):

Calories: 160

Carbs: 19,4 g
Fat: 8 g
Fiber: 4,7 g
Protein: 5,7 g

7.7 - Lemon Spinach Mix

Preparation time: 10 minutes
Cooking time: 15 minutes
Servings: **2**

Ingredients:

- 6 mushrooms, chopped
- A handful cherry tomatoes, cut in halves
- 3 handfuls spinach, torn
- 1 teaspoon ghee
- 2 tablespoons extra virgin olive oil
- 1 small red onion, sliced
- ½ teaspoon lemon rind, diced
- 1 garlic clove, minced
- A pinch of sea salt
- Black pepper to taste
- A pinch of nutmeg
- A drizzle of lemon juice

Directions:

1. Heat up a pan with the ghee over medium-high heat, add mushrooms, stir, cook for 4 minutes and transfer them to a plate.
2. Heat up the same pan with the olive oil over medium-high heat, add onion, stir and cook for 3 minutes.
3. Add tomatoes, a pinch of sea salt, pepper, lemon rind, nutmeg, and garlic, stir and cook for 3 minutes more.
4. Add spinach, stir and cook for 2-3 minutes.
5. Add lemon juice at the end, stir gently, transfer to plates and serve with mushrooms on top.

Nutritional Values (Per Serving):

Calories: 178

Carbs: 9,9 g
Fat: 16,5 g
Fiber: 2,3 g
Protein: 3,3 g

7.8 - Carrots and Pineapple Sauce

Preparation time: 10 minutes
Cooking time: 15 minutes
Servings: **4**

Ingredients:

- 1 pound carrots, sliced
- 1 tablespoon coconut oil
- 1 tablespoon ghee
- ½ cup pineapple juice
- 1 teaspoon ginger, grated
- ½ tablespoon maple syrup
- ½ teaspoon nutmeg
- 1 tablespoon parsley, chopped

Directions:

---

1. Heat a pan with the ghee and the oil over medium-high heat, add ginger, stir and cook for 2 minutes.
2. Add carrots, stir and cook for 5 minutes.
3. Add pineapple juice, maple syrup and nutmeg, stir and cook for 5 minutes more.
4. Add parsley, stir, cook for 3 minutes, divide between plates and serve.

Nutritional Values (Per Serving):

Calories: 130

Carbs: 17,4 g
Fat: 6,8 g
Fiber: 3 g
Protein: 1,1 g

Preparation time: 10 minutes
Cooking time: 10 minutes
Servings: **4**

Ingredients:

- 1 pound watercress, chopped
- ¼ cup olive oil
- 1 garlic clove, cut in halves
- 1 small shallot, peeled, cooked and chopped ¼ cup hazelnuts, chopped Black pepper to taste
- ¼ cup pine nuts

Directions:

1. Heat up a pan with the oil over medium heat, add garlic clove halves, cook for 2 minutes and discard.
2. Heat up the pan with the garlic oil again over medium heat, add hazelnuts and pine nuts, stir and cook for 6 minutes.
3. Add shallots, black pepper to taste and watercress, stir, cook for 2 minutes, divide between plates and serve right away.

Nutritional Values (Per Serving):

Calories: 220

Carbs: 2,9 g
Fat: 21,8 g
Fiber: 2,1 g
Protein: 5,3 g

7.10 - Anchovy Stuffed Peppers

Preparation time: 10 minutes
Cooking time: 40 minutes
Servings: **4**

Ingredients:

- ¼ cup ghee, melted
- 6 colored bell peppers
- 1 garlic head, cloves peeled and chopped
- 10 anchovy fillets
- 15 walnuts

Directions:

1. Put the peppers on a lined baking sheet, place under a preheated broiler, cook for 20 minutes and leave them to cool down.
2. Heat up a pan with the ghee over low heat, add garlic, stir and cook for 10 minutes.
3. Grind walnuts in a coffee grinder and add this powder to the pan.
4. Also add anchovy and stir well.
5. Peel burnt skin off peppers, discard tops, cut in halves and remove skins.
6. Divide pepper halves on plates, divide anchovy mix on them and serve.

Nutritional Values (Per Serving):

Calories: 358

Carbs: 12,9 g
Fat: 31,3 g
Fiber: 5,1 g
Protein: 11,8 g

Salads

8.1 - Basil Turkey and Tomato Salad

Preparation time: 10 minutes
Cooking time: 0 minutes
Servings: **4**

Ingredients:

- For the salad dressing:
- 1 tablespoon basil, chopped
- 1 teaspoon rosemary, chopped
- ½ cup avocado homemade mayonnaise
- 1 garlic clove, minced
- A pinch of sea salt
- Black pepper to taste
- 1 teaspoon lemon juice
- For the salad:
- 6 baby lettuce heads, chopped
- 1 cup cherry tomatoes, halved
- ½ pound turkey meat, cooked and chopped 2 green onions, chopped

Directions:

1. In a bowl, mix basil with rosemary, mayo, garlic, lemon juice, a pinch of salt and black pepper and whisk well.
2. In a salad bowl, mix lettuce with tomatoes, green onions and turkey meat.
3. Add salad dressing, toss to coat and serve.

Nutritional Values (Per Serving):

Calories: 252

Carbs: 6,5 g
Fat: 18 g
Fiber: 3 g
Protein: 18,5 g

8.2 - Balsamic Cabbage Salad

Preparation time: 10 minutes
Cooking time: 6 minutes
Servings: **4**

Ingredients:

- 1 red cabbage head, shredded
- 2 tablespoons olive oil
- A pinch of sea salt
- Black pepper to taste
- ¼ cup balsamic vinegar
- ½ teaspoon oregano, dried
- 1 yellow onion, chopped
- 1 tablespoon maple syrup
- 2 figs, cut into quarters
- A handful oregano, chopped

Directions:

1. In a bowl mix cabbage with a pinch of salt and some black pepper, stir well and leave aside.
2. Heat up a pan with half of the oil over medium heat, add onion, stir and cook for 4 minutes.
3. Add dried oregano and vinegar, stir, cook for 5 minutes and take off heat.
4. Add maple syrup, some black pepper and stir well.
5. In a salad bowl, mix squeezed cabbage with onions mix, figs and the rest of the oil, toss to coat and serve with fresh oregano on top.

Nutritional Values (Per Serving):

Calories: 156

Carbs: 23,4 g
Fat: 7,3 g
Fiber: 6,1 g
Protein: 2,9 g

8.3 - Prosciutto, Cabbage and Pecan Salad

Preparation time: 10 minutes
Cooking time: 15 minutes
Servings: **4**

Ingredients:

- 1 purple cabbage head, cut into thin strips
- 4 prosciutto slices
- 1 red onion, thinly sliced
- 1 green apple, cored and chopped
- ½ cup pecans, toasted
- A handful watercress
- ½ cup olive oil
- 1 garlic clove, minced
- ¼ cup balsamic vinegar
- 1 teaspoon honey
- ½ teaspoon mustard
- A pinch of sea salt
- Black pepper to taste

Directions:

1. Place prosciutto slices on a lined baking sheet, place in the oven at 350 degrees F and cook for 15 minutes.
2. Leave prosciutto to cool down and chop it.
3. In a salad bowl mix cabbage with prosciutto, onion, apple pieces, watercress and pecans and toss.
4. In another bowl, mix olive oil with honey, vinegar, garlic, mustard, a pinch of salt and black pepper and whisk well.
5. Drizzle this over your salad and serve.

Nutritional Values (Per Serving):

Calories: 589

Carbs: 26,2 g
Fat: 40,9 g
Fiber: 7,7 g
Protein: 33,4 g

Preparation time: 10 minutes
Cooking time: 0 minutes
Servings: **3**

Ingredients:

- 1 lettuce head, chopped
- A handful kale, chopped
- A handful steamed broccoli
- A handful walnuts, chopped
- 8 cherry tomatoes, halved
- A handful radishes, chopped
- 1 tablespoon lemon juice
- 8 dates, chopped
- A drizzle of olive oil

Directions:

1. In a salad bowl, mix lettuce with kale, broccoli, walnuts, tomatoes, radishes and dates.
2. In smaller bowl, mix lemon juice with olive oil and whisk well.
3. Add this to salad, toss to coat and serve.

Nutritional Values (Per Serving):

Calories: 771

Carbs: 112,4 g
Fat: 35,2 g
Fiber: 36,2 g
Protein: 21,4 g

8.5 - Chicken and Olives Salad

Preparation time: 10 minutes
Cooking time: 0 minutes
Servings: **1**

Ingredients:

- 1 chicken breast, cooked and sliced
- 1 medium lettuce head, chopped
- 1 sweet potato, boiled and cubed
- 1 tablespoon pumpkin seeds
- 6 black olives, pitted and chopped
- 1 tablespoon olive oil
- 1 tablespoon balsamic vinegar

Directions:

1. In a salad bowl, mix chicken breast slices with lettuce, sweet potato, pumpkin seeds, olives, olive oil and balsamic vinegar, stir well and serve right away.

Nutritional Values (Per Serving):

Calories: 760

Carbs: 43,1 g
Fat: 30,4 g
Fiber: 8,4 g
Protein: 78,3 g

8.6 - Shrimp and Apple Salad

Preparation time: 10 minutes
Cooking time: 0 minutes
Servings: **3**

Ingredients:

- 1 green apple, cored and chopped
- 2 cups shrimp, peeled, deveined, cooked and chopped
- 3 eggs, hard-boiled, peeled and chopped
- 1 small red onion, chopped
- ¼ cup Dijon mustard
- 4 celery stalks, chopped
- 1 tablespoon olive oil
- 2 tablespoons vinegar
- ½ teaspoon thyme, chopped
- ½ teaspoon parsley, chopped
- ½ teaspoon basil, chopped
- A pinch of sea salt
- Black pepper to taste

Directions:

1. In a big salad bowl, mix apple pieces with shrimp, eggs, onion and celery and stir.
2. In another bowl, mix mustard with oil, vinegar, thyme, parsley, basil, a pinch of salt and black pepper and whisk well.
3. Add this to your salad, toss well and serve.

Nutritional Values (Per Serving):

Calories: 389

Carbs: 17,6 g
Fat: 13,2 g
Fiber: 3,4 g
Protein: 48,9 g

8.7 - Shrimp and Turkey Salad

Preparation time: 10 minutes
Cooking time: 4 minutes
Servings: **4**

Ingredients:

- 5 oz turkey meat, cooked and chopped
- 1 tablespoon olive oil
- 1 pound shrimp, peeled and deveined
- 1 teaspoon garlic powder
- A pinch of sea salt
- Black pepper to taste
- 6 cups romaine lettuce leaves, chopped
- 4 eggs, hard-boiled, peeled and chopped
- 1-pint cherry tomatoes, halved
- 1 avocado, pitted, peeled and chopped
- For the vinaigrette:
- 1 garlic clove, minced
- 2 tablespoons Paleo mayonnaise
- 2 tablespoon vinegar
- 3 tablespoons avocado oil

Directions:

1. In a bowl mix garlic with mayo, vinegar and avocado oil, whisk well and leave aside for now.
2. Heat up a pan with the olive oil over medium-high heat, add shrimp, season with a pinch of salt, some black pepper and garlic powder, cook for 2 minutes, flip, cook for 2 minutes more and transfer them to a salad bowl.

3. Add tomatoes, avocado pieces, lettuce leaves, turkey and egg pieces and stir.
4. Add the vinaigrette you've made earlier, toss to coat and serve.

Nutritional Values (Per Serving):

Calories: 561

carbs13,2 g
Fat: 37,2 g
Fiber: 5,1 g
Protein: 44 g

8.8 - Lime Veggie Noodle Salad

Preparation time: 15 minutes
Cooking time: 0 minutes
Servings: **4**

Ingredients:

- 3 carrots, thinly sliced with a spiralizer
- 2 cucumbers, thinly sliced with a spiralizer
- 1 green onion, sliced
- 1 tablespoon sesame seeds
- 2 tablespoons lime juice
- A pinch of sea salt
- 2 tablespoons balsamic vinegar
- Black pepper to taste
- 2 tablespoons extra virgin olive oil

Directions:

1. In a salad bowl, mix cucumbers with green onion and carrots.
2. In a small bowl, mix vinegar with olive oil, lime juice, a pinch of sea salt, and pepper to taste and stir well.
3. Pour this over salad, toss to coat and keep in the fridge until you serve it.

Calories: 117

Carbs: 11,2 g
Fat: 8,3 g
Fiber: 2,3 g
Protein: 1,9 g

8.9 - Cabbage and Mayo Salad

Preparation time: 10 minutes
Cooking time: 0 minutes
Servings: **4**

Ingredients:

- 2 cup red cabbage, chopped
- 4 cups Brussels sprouts, shredded
- 2 tablespoons lemon juice
- 4 tablespoons balsamic vinegar
- ¼ cup Paleo mayonnaise
- 1 red apple, cored and chopped
- 2 celery sticks, chopped
- ¼ cup walnuts, chopped
- A pinch of sea salt
- Black pepper to taste

Directions:

1. In a salad bowl, mix cabbage with Brussels sprouts, apple, celery and walnuts.
2. In another bowl, mix lemon juice with vinegar, a pinch of salt, black pepper and mayo and whisk well.
3. Add this to salad, toss to coat and serve.

Calories: 242

Carbs: 19,8 g
Fat: 17,6 g
Fiber: 6,6 g
Protein: 5,8 g

8.10 - Chicken and Nuts Salad

Preparation time: 10 minutes
Cooking time: 0 minutes
Servings: **2**

Ingredients:

- 1 and ½ tablespoons vinegar
- 3 tablespoons olive oil
- 1 teaspoon thyme, dried
- 2 tablespoons macadamia nuts, chopped
- A pinch of sea salt
- Black pepper to taste
- ¾ cup chicken, cooked and shredded
- 3 tablespoons onion, chopped
- ¼ cup carrot, grated
- 4 radishes, chopped
- ½ cup red cabbage, shredded
- ½ cup green cabbage, shredded

Directions:

1. In a salad bowl, mix chicken with macadamia nuts, carrot, onion, radishes, green and red cabbage.
2. In a bowl, mix vinegar with oil, a pinch of salt, black pepper and thyme and whisk well.
3. Add this to salad, toss to coat and serve.

Nutritional Values (Per Serving):

Calories: 398

Carbs: 5,7 g
Fat: 29,3 g
Fiber: 2,2 g
Protein: 16,5 g

Desserts

9.1 - Berry and Dates Cheesecake

Preparation time: 2 hours and 10 minutes
Cooking time: 0 minutes
Servings: **4**

Ingredients:

- For the crust:
- ½ cup pecans
- ½ cup macadamia nuts
- ½ cup dates
- ½ cup walnuts
- For the filling:
- 1 cup date paste
- 3 cups cashews, soaked for 3 hours
- ½ cup almond milk
- 2 cups strawberries
- ¾ cup coconut oil
- ¼ cup lime juice
- Sliced limes for serving
- Sliced strawberries for serving

Directions:

1. Put nuts, walnuts, dates and pecans in a food processor and blend well.
2. Put 3 spoons of crust mix each part of a muffin tin, press well and leave aside for now.
3. Put cashews, strawberries, date paste, lime juice, almond milk and coconut oil in the food processor and blend well.

4. Put 3 spoons of filling mix on top of crust mix, place in the freezer and keep for 2 hours.
5. Transfer cheesecakes on a platter, top with strawberries and limes and serve.

Nutritional Values (Per Serving):

Calories: 1569

Carbs: 99,9 g
Fat: 130,6 g
Fiber: 15,4 g
Protein: 25,7 g

9.2 - Maple Ice Cream

Preparation time: 2 hours
Cooking time: 3 minutes
Servings: **8**

Ingredients:

- 1 tablespoon arrowroot powder
- 2 cans coconut milk
- ¼ teaspoon vanilla beans
- 1 tablespoon water
- 1/3 cup pure maple syrup
- 1/3 cup coconut nectar

Directions:

1. Fill 1/3 of a bowl with ice cubes, place another bowl on top and leave aside for now.
2. Pour coconut milk in a saucepan, reserve 2 tablespoons, put them in a bowl, mix with arrowroot starch and stir well.
3. Add arrowroot mix of coconut milk to the saucepan and stir.
4. Also add vanilla beans, maple syrup and coconut nectar, stir well, place on stove and heat up over medium heat.
5. Stir well, bring to a boil, boil for 2 minutes, take off heat and pour into the bowl you've placed over the ice.
6. Add water, stir well and leave aside for 1 hour and 30 minutes.
7. Pour this into your ice cream machine and turn on.
8. Pour into a container, place in the freezer and leave it there for 20 minutes.

9. Serve right away!

Calories: 151

Carbs: 6 g
Fat: 14,5 g
Fiber: 1,5 g
Protein: 1,4 g

9.3 - Lemon Berry Mix

Preparation time: 5 minutes
Cooking time: 15 minutes
Servings: **4**

Ingredients:

- 2 tablespoons lemon juice
- 1 and ½ tablespoons maple syrup
- 1 and ½ tablespoons balsamic vinegar
- 1 tablespoon olive oil
- 1 pound strawberries, halved
- 1 and ½ cups blueberries
- ¼ cup basil leaves, torn

Directions:

1. In a saucepan, mix lemon juice with maple syrup and vinegar, bring to a boil at a medium-high temperature, simmer for 15 minutes, add oil, stir and leave aside for 2 minutes.
2. In a bowl, mix blueberries with strawberries and lemon vinaigrette, toss to coat, sprinkle basil on top and serve!

Nutritional Values (Per Serving):

Calories: 135

Carbs: 25,7 g
Fat: 4,2 g
Fiber: 4,3 g
Protein: 1,4 g

9.4 - Pineapple Cake

Preparation time: 3 hours and 15 minutes
Cooking time: 0 minutes
Servings: **6**

Ingredients:

- For the cashew frosting:
- 2 tablespoons lemon juice
- 2 cups cashews, soaked
- 2 tablespoons coconut oil, melted
- 1/3 cup maple syrup
- Water
- For the cake:
- 1 cup pineapple, dried and chopped
- 2 carrots, chopped
- 1 and ½ cups coconut flour
- 1 cup dates, pitted
- ½ cup dry coconut
- ½ teaspoon cinnamon

Directions:

1. In a blender, mix cashews with lemon juice, coconut oil, maple syrup and some apple, pulse well, transfer to a bowl and leave aside for now.
2. Put carrots in a food processor and pulse a few times.
3. Add flour, dates, pineapple, coconut and cinnamon and pulse well again.
4. Pour half of this mix into a springform pan and spread evenly.
5. Add 1/3 of the frosting and spread.

6. Add the rest of the cake mix and the rest of the frosting.
7. Place in the freezer and keep until it's hard enough.
8. Cut and serve.

Nutritional Values (Per Serving):

Calories: 628

Carbs: 80,8 g
Fat: 31,9 g
Fiber: 20,3 g
Protein: 13,3 g

9.5 - Coconut and Banana Pancakes

Preparation time: 15 minutes
Cooking time: 20 minutes
Servings: **4**

Ingredients:

- ¼ cup coconut milk
- 1 banana, peeled and mashed
- 4 eggs
- 1 teaspoon vanilla extract
- 1 and ½ cups hazelnut meal
- 2 tablespoons coconut flour
- ½ teaspoon baking soda
- Ghee for cooking
- For the sauce:
- 2 tablespoons coconut oil
- 1 tablespoon lemon juice
- 2 blood oranges, peeled and sliced
- Juice from 1 blood orange
- 2 teaspoons stevia
- 1 vanilla bean

Directions:

1. Heat up a pan with the coconut oil over medium heat, add orange juice, lemon juice, stevia and vanilla bean, bring to a boil and simmer for 15 minutes stirring from time to time.
2. In a bowl, mix eggs with vanilla extract and coconut milk and stir.

3. Add mashed banana, coconut flour, baking soda and hazelnut meal and stir well.
4. Heat up a pan with the ghee over medium heat, spoon ¼ cup pancake mix, spread a bit, cook for 3 minutes on one side, flip, cook for 1 more minute and transfer to a plate.
5. Repeat this with the rest of the batter and serve pancakes with orange slices on the side and with the orange sauce on top.

Nutritional Values (Per Serving):

Calories: 696

Carbs: 41,4 g
Fat: 56,5 g
Fiber: 12,7 g
Protein: 17 g

9.6 - Chia and Maple Ramekins

Preparation time: 10 minutes
Cooking time: 1 hour
Servings: **6**

Ingredients:

- 1 and ½ cups pumpkin puree
- 2/3 cup maple syrup
- 1 cup coconut milk
- 2 tablespoons chia seeds ground and mixed with 5 tablespoons water 1/4 teaspoon baking soda
- 2 tablespoons lemon juice
- 2 teaspoons pumpkin pie spice
- A pinch of salt
- 1 teaspoon cinnamon
- ½ teaspoon vanilla
- Pumpkin seeds for serving

Directions:

1. In a bowl, mix pumpkin puree with coconut milk, maple syrup, chia seeds mixed with water, baking soda, lemon juice, pumpkin pie spice, a pinch of salt, cinnamon and vanilla and stir well using a kitchen mixer.
2. Pour this into small ramekins, arrange them on a baking tray filled half way with hot water, place in the oven at 325 degrees F and bake for 1 hour.
3. Take custards out of the oven, leave them to cool down and serve with pumpkin seeds on top.

Nutritional Values (Per Serving):

Calories: 253

Carbs: 32,1 g
Fat: 13,8 g
Fiber: 4 g
Protein: 3,5 g

Indexes in Alphabetical Order

Index of Recipes

A

B

C

P

S

T

V

W

Z

Index of Ingredients

A

B

C

V

W

Z

CPSIA information can be obtained
at www.ICGtesting.com
Printed in the USA
LVHW050211050621
689455LV00025B/1813